Care Worker's Handbook

March 2014

E.W. Ndungu

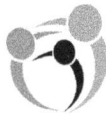

Bettercare Skills Ltd

First edition published by Bettercare Skills Ltd
89 Wilkins Road, Oxford OX4 2JB, UK
Company Registration No. 8380433

ISBN: 978-0-9576004-6-1

Printed and bound in Great Britain by
Lightning Source UK Ltd,
Chapter House, Pitfield, Kiln Farm,
Milton Keynes MK11 3LW

Note on copyright and permissions
In the case of any material that has been reproduced from a
published source, the author has made every effort to obtain
permission from the copyright holder(s); if she has unknowingly
breached anyone's copyright she will be glad to amend the text
accordingly in subsequent reprints.

Author's note
The information provided here is for general guidance only.
All organisations have their own procedures in place.

Content	Care Worker's Sign	Manager's Sign	Date
Introduction			
Communication			
Confidentiality			
Challenging Behaviour			
Care Provision			
Health and Safety			
Medication			
Moving & Handling			
Food Safety			
Infection Control			
Fire Safety			
Equality and Diversity			
Abuse – Safeguarding of Vulnerable Adults			
Lone Working			
Violence at Work			
Record Keeping			

Care Worker's Handbook

This handbook has been developed to support you and is a self-managed induction handbook, to provide you with the guidance and key points of policies and procedures that you should follow through your work in health and social care and what you need to know

Your knowledge and understanding for this handbook relates to legal requirements and codes of practice applicable to the scope of your work and others with whom you work; the nature of the work you will be undertaking; your role and level of responsibility within the organisation (e.g. whether you have responsibility to support the work of others); the service users and the key people in their lives.

This handbook provides you with that information; however, the information provided here does not replace policies.

Reading gives you an understanding but working gives you the experience when you apply the knowledge you have read. It will help you avoid trial and error in your work and empower you to carry out safe practice.

E.W. Ndungu
Oxford, March 2014

Types of Services

There are different types of services that provide individualised support packages, these include;

Individual tenancies - With this type of tenancies the individual service user is responsible for the entire house with the support of the service provider in connection with Housing Associations.

Specialist care homes for people with high support needs, including profound physical disabilities, complex or challenging behaviour

Adapted flats for one or two people with multiple occupancy buildings

Adapted bungalows within a serviced site, to provide accommodation on an individual basis

Supported living models for up to four people sharing a tenancy

Outreach and domiciliary enables people to live in their own homes or with their families and actively engage in the community where they live, attending college, working and developing leisure activities

Registered Homes provide people with personal care and support, with a range of activities of their own choosing; along with minimal possible structure to offer people the security they need

Personalised Supported **Living** is designed and managed to provide people with independent lifestyles that meet their own aspirations, as members of their local communities

Flexible Respite centres offer service user one to two weeks planned and regular breaks from their usual care environment.

Terms and definitions of the key words and concepts used in health and social care settings.

Care provider – The organisation responsible for providing care services; the owner/management of the home/project

Interaction – The action and influence exerted by people on one another –how we behave has an effect on how other people respond to us

Residential setting – A 'home' set up to provide care and a place to live

Service setting – Where the social care is provided – this will affect the way that care is organised

Service user group – Broad description of groups of people cared for – for example, older people or adults with learning disabilities

Staff – This may be regular members of staff, or members of agency staff temporarily working in the organisation in a particular service setting

Active Support- is working in a way that recognises that people have the right to take part in the activities and relationships of everyday life as independently as they can, and so give them support by helping only with what they really cannot manage to do for themselves.

Service user – The people being helped by the service – often this is not just the people being cared for, but also their families and friends. The term 'service users' is used because the focus is on people with a range of needs who are using the services

Key people – Those people who are key to an individual's (service user) health and social well-being, they include: family; friends; carers; advocates and others with whom the service user has a supportive relationship

Practice – Practice covers every aspect of the work you do including your skills, knowledge, attitudes and behaviour. It also involves experiences and personal beliefs that might affect your practice

Feedback – Comments about your strengths or areas that need developing, they are useful for improving your practice and could be communicated: verbally; in written form; electronically; or in other forms of communication.

Development opportunities – opportunities that enable you to develop and work more effectively this could include: training; educational programmes; reading material; personal and professional support.

Personal and Professional Development – Knowledge and practice of any type that will enable you to develop within your job role both as a person and as a care worker

Information could include: service plans; care needs assessments; records and reports.

Risks could include the possibility of: danger, damage and destruction to the environment and goods; injury and harm to people; self-injurious behaviour and abuse.

Introduction

Competent practice is a combination of the application of skills and knowledge informed by values and ethics. This details the knowledge and understanding required to carry out safe practice in a care environment. During your induction it is important to acquire the skills necessary in relation to expectations and requirements of your job role. You need to show that you know, understand and can apply in practice:

Values - These include;

- legal and organisational requirements on equality, diversity, discrimination and rights when working with service users and others to improve your knowledge and skills
- dilemmas and conflicts that you may face in your workplace

You need to show that you know, understand and can apply in practice:

Current legislation, organisational policies and procedures for;

o Confidentiality - data protection, including recording, reporting, storage, security and sharing of information with other organisations and agencies.

o Health and safety – maintaining safety at work

o Medication – administration, documentation and storage

o Risk assessment and management

o Dealing with comments and complaints

o Promoting the well-being and protection of service users – safeguarding of vulnerable adults o   Care planning – provision and delivery of care

Service user complaints

What is complaint?

"Complaint is an expression of dissatisfaction, however made, about the standard or quality of service, action or lack of action, by an organisation or its staff affecting an individual or a group of individuals in receipt of a service provided by the organisation".

All organisations actively seek the opinion and comments of service users with regard to the suitability and professionalism of the services requested and supplied. As a care worker, you should recognise service users' rights to complain if they so wish. This should not be met with hostility but it is your role to explain carefully to a service user how best to make their complaint by giving them the information that they need. It is essential that this information is relevant, up to date and provided in a way that is appropriate to the service user

Independent Advice

Organisations always try to resolve complaints informally. However, should a complainant feel it is important that they get independent advice before proceeding with a formal complaint; support the service user to contact local agencies that may be able offer assistance, these include;

- Welfare Right Services
- Citizens Advice Bureau
- Law Centre
- A Solicitor

COMMUNICATION

Communication has been included in this induction standard because it is important that care workers have basic skills in communication before working alone with service users.

What is communication?

Communication, as defined by most sources, is the process of conveying information from a sender to a receiver through the use of a medium or channel that is understood by the sender and receiver. While this describes communication in a very general sense, communication is far more than simply conveying information. Communication is how we exchange our thoughts, feelings or ideas; how we assign and convey meaning in an attempt to create a shared understanding; how we utilise signals or words to produce a desired effect (eHow.com)

Communication is, therefore, putting the right emphasis on and utilising all our senses in listening, seeing, hearing, understanding and then digesting the facts in a systematic manner. Only after the processing of all available information is done by the brain and the ideas are assimilated properly can we think up a proper response.

Importance of effective communication in care environment

Effective communication and interaction play an important role in the work of all health and social care professionals. For example, care professionals need to be able to use a range of communication and interaction skills in order to:

- work inclusively with people of different ages and diverse backgrounds;

- respond appropriately to the variety of care-related problems and individual needs of people who use care services;

- enable people to feel relaxed and secure enough to talk openly

- ask sensitive and difficult questions, and obtain information about matters that might be very personal and sensitive;

- obtain clear, accurate information about a person's problems, symptoms or concerns;

- give others information about care-related issues in a clear, confident and competent way.

    As a care worker you should understand the language needs and communication preferences of the service user with whom you work. You should be able to;

    Communicate using their preferred methods of communication and language,

- use the individual's preferred spoken language;

- the use of signs; symbols; pictures; writing; objects of reference;

- Communication passports – (communication passport is a small book or folder which contains information about the details of a service user who want to tell others about themselves. It contains, the person's names and where they live; how the person communicates and how to communicate with them; things that the person likes and dislikes; any medical condition, e.g. epilepsy, what medication they take and how to support them in case of a fit.

- Human and technological aids in communication – language signers and interpreters, telephone amplifiers, hearing loops, etc.

Main elements of nonverbal communication

What is nonverbal communication?

Nonverbal communication is behaviour that creates or represents meaning. It includes facial expressions, body movements, and gestures. In other words, nonverbal communication is talking without speaking a word

While nonverbal communication and behaviour can vary considerably between cultures, the facial expressions for happiness, sadness, anger and fear are similar throughout the world. You should be aware of the meaning of nonverbal communication and behaviour, such as;

1. *Proximity* - means being near or close to someone or something, for example if a service user stands next to the kettle they could be asking for a cup of tea.

2. *Body language* is a form of nonverbal communication, which consists of body posture, gestures, facial expressions, and eye movements by which attitudes and feelings are communicated. E.g. waving your arms around can indicate you are excited or agitated about something.
3. *Facial expression* - Facial expression is the movement of the face that express a person's feelings; for example, wide eyes is a show of surprise, interest in someone or recognition.

4. *Eye contact* - is a meeting of the eyes between two individuals. It is important to remember that good eye contact does not mean staring fixedly into someone's eyes

5. *Gesture* - are planned movements and signals using parts of the body like hands, head etc.

6. *Touch or contact* - Touch can be used to communicate affection, familiarity, sympathy and other emotions to another person. E.g. A touch on a service user's elbow with sight impairment to guide them

7. *Appearance* - Our choice of colour, clothing, hairstyles and other factors affecting appearance are also considered a means of nonverbal communication

8. *Signs* - There are certain common gestures made using body language, facial expressions that most people automatically recognise, for example:

- a wave of the hand can mean hello or goodbye;
- thumbs up can mean that all is well;
- using fingers can indicate numeric amounts.

9. *Symbols* - A symbol is an item or image that is used to represent something that communicates information.

10. *Hand movement* - There are three main uses of nonverbal communication using hand movement that is greetings, shaking hands and salute

11. *Head movement* - People may use head movements to reinforce or modify what they are saying. For example, someone may nod their heads vigorously when saying 'Yes', to emphasise that they agree with another person, or shake their head to indicate that they disagree.

12. *Posture* - is the way we sit or stand, and it is important as it convey messages. Good, straight posture indicates confidence. It tells the audience that you are in control. It conveys the message that you have confidence in your competence.

Pictures - *o*f all forms communicate messages; a picture of a plate and spoon will signify that it's time for food.

Objects - may have a particular meaning for a person (e.g. a special ring or ornament) while others may represent the same thing to lots of people, e.g. a cup may be associated with tea or coffee.

Verbal skills to overcome communication barriers

What is verbal communication?

Verbal communication is an act of conveying messages, ideas, information, or feelings through the use of mouth, the key components being words, sound, speaking, and language.

Using verbal skills effectively can help overcome barriers that might be preventing effective communication. Some of the skills needed when communicating verbally with service users or colleagues include the following;

Assertion

Being assertive means that you express yourself effectively and stand up for your point of view, while also respecting the rights and beliefs of others. Assertion helps people to communicate their needs, feelings and thoughts in a clear confident way while taking into account the feelings of others and respecting their right to an opinion as well.

How to be assertive

- *Be polite:* state the nature of the problem, how it affects you, how you feel about it and what you want to happen. Make it clear that you see the other person's point of view and be prepared to compromise if it leads to what you want.

- *Control your emotions:* emotions such as anger or tearfulness can hinder effective communication. Therefore, be calm and authoritative in your interactions with others. You need to be clear and concise.

- *Be prepared* to defend your position and be able to say no. This won't cause offence if it is said firmly and calmly.

- *Use questions such* as, 'How can we solve this problem?' Use the 'broken record' technique where you just keep repeating your statement softly, calmly and persistently.

- Use body language that shows you are relaxed, e.g. make firm, direct eye contact with relaxed facial features and use open hand gestures.

Paraphrasing

Paraphrasing means repeating back something a person has just said in a different way to make sure you have understood the message. For example, if someone says, 'I have been sick since Sunday' you could respond by saying, 'you have been unwell now for four days then?'

Closed questions

Closed questions are questions that can be answered with either a single word or short phrase, for example, 'Do you like sprouts?' could be answered, 'No' or, 'No, I can't stand them.'

o Closed questions give facts, are easy and quick to answer and keep control of the conversation.

o Closed questions are useful as an opening question, such as 'Are you feeling better?', for testing understanding, such as, 'So you want to go on the pill?' and for bringing a conversation to an end, such as, 'So that's your final decision?'

Open questions

Open questions are questions that give a longer answer, for example, 'Why don't you like sprouts?' might be answered by, 'I haven't liked the taste or smell of them since I was made to eat them every time when I was a child...'

- Open questions hand control of the conversation to the person you are speaking to.

- They ask the person to think and reflect, give opinions and express their feelings.

- They are useful as a follow-up to a closed question, to find out more information, to help someone realise or face their problems and to show concern about them.

Clarification

- Clarification means to make something clear and understandable, using a form of communication suitable for the people you are working with.

Summarising

- Summarising means to sum up what has been said in a short, clear way.

Good practice of effective communication you should know

Active listening

What is active listening?

Active listening is a way of listening and responding that focuses the attention on the speaker

The process of active listening involves:

- allowing the person talking time to explain without interrupting;

- giving encouragement by smiling, nodding and making encouraging remarks such as, 'That's interesting' and 'Really?'

- asking questions for clarification, such as, 'Can you explain that again please? 'to avoid misunderstanding

- showing empathy by making comments such as, 'That must be making life really hard for you';

- looking interested by maintaining eye contact and not looking at your watch every three minutes;

- not being distracted by anything, such as a ringing mobile phone.

- summarising to check that you have understood the other person; you can do this by paraphrasing, 'So what you mean is …?'

Written communication skills

Written communication can be defined as any type of interaction that makes use of the written word. It is one of the two main types of communication, along with oral/spoken communication.

It has three elements; structure (the way the material is laid out), style (the way the material is written) and content (what the material written is about).

- Care workers should to be able to communicate well with the written word. This could be by writing daily   reports and record-keeping of finances, a record of a service user's condition and support needs

- Care workers should to be able to use different ways of presenting information, such as letters, memoranda, emails, reports or filling forms.

- Writing should be legible so that the person the information is intended for can actually read and understand it, and the language used is appropriate.

CONFIDENTIALITY

What is confidentiality?

Confidentiality is the preservation of secret information concerning the client which is disclosed in the professional relationship. Confidentiality is based on a basic right of the client; it is an ethical obligation of the caseworker and is necessary for the effective casework service. The client's rights, however, is not absolute. Moreover, the client's secret is often shared with other professional persons within the agency and in other agencies; the obligation then binds all equally. (Biestek (1961) quoted in Thomson (2000).

Importance of Confidentiality

- Confidentiality is crucial in enabling a service user to feel comfortable enough to discuss sensitive personal matters. It is essential they feel they are able to speak freely without the information they provide being available to people outside their care and that health and social care professionals are trustworthy.

- Personal information disclosed to you during the course of your work should be treated as confidential and should only be disclosed with the consent of the person concerned, unless an emergency makes it impossible to obtain their consent.

- You may disclose information to those with direct need for information (such as healthcare professional, care managers and your line manager). Relatives, neighbours and friends are not entitled to receive confidential information

Elements of good practice

- Avoid passing on confidential information during informal conversations on service users or colleagues.

- Write up records in a way that keeps all service users' information confidential from each other. If you have to refer to another service user in another's daily notes remember to use initials.

- Never promise to keep a secret (remember, it may put someone at risk). It is important to remind the service users that should there be a situation of risk, you (the care worker) will have to share the information with the service manager. If significant information is not passed on to a service manager or team leader, there may be several risks:

  o The care worker may find themselves compromised.

  o There may be a failure to meet the service user's needs because others are unable to take the necessary action.

  o The service user may be at risk as secrets may lead to an inappropriate relationship.

  o Other people may be at risk because the information was not shared.

- Service users should, where appropriate, be asked to give consent if information is to be shared.

- Files or records should be stored in a safe place and not removed from the offices where they are kept.

  The following elements of good practice should apply to sharing information of personal nature without consent outside of the team environment in order to:

- facilitate the delivery of corporate services, e.g. income recovery;

- ensure consistency in support, progression and recovery when a service user transfers between services;

- enable effective internal audit and evidence of care being given;

- reduce the potential risk to health, safety and well-being of service users and staff;

- for monitoring and review purposes to ensure compliance with standards, legislation and good practice

Data Protection

The Data Protection Act (1998) is the legislation that provides a framework that governs the processing of information that identifies living individuals.

Personal data is information relating to an individual from whom they can be identified, e.g. name, address, tax details or national insurance number, ethnic origin, health status, income support needs, tenancy history etc., which is held on file, electronically and /or in hard copy. Processing this information is subject to the Data Protection Act 1998.

- The processing of data includes holding, obtaining, recording, using and disclosing of information and the Act applies to all forms of media, including paper and images.

- Data Protection applies to confidential patient information but is far wider in its scope, in that it also covers staff records

Storage and transportation of information

- Information should be stored in an area that ensures that neither other service users, members of the public or unauthorised members of staff can gain access to them.

- Where information is stored in areas that do not have 24-hour staff presence, it should be stored in an area that can be securely locked when the premises are unstaffed.

- If information needs to be transported from one care setting area to another, it is the responsibility of the staff member to ensure that at no point could the information be accessed by unauthorised individuals.

- It is staff responsibility to ensure that any information is stored safely and securely whilst in transit.

- All computer-held information should be password protected and only accessible by authorised users.

CHALLENGING BEHAVIOUR

What is challenging behaviour?

The term challenging behaviour has been defined as 'culturally abnormal behaviour(s) of such intensity, frequency or duration that the physical safety of the person or others is likely to be placed in serious jeopardy, or behaviour which is likely to seriously limit use of, or result in to a person being denied access to, ordinary community facilities. (Emerson, 1995, pp. 4–5)

Causes of Challenging Behaviour

Communication factors may include;

Communication difficulties

Being nonverbal, hearing loss, unclear communication, insufficient vocabulary or means of expression, difficulties understanding communication of others and lacking the communication and emotional skills to convey what they need.

For people with autism who have no other way to communicate that they are experiencing sensory overload, difficulty with transitions, or unable to communicate needs or wants, challenging behaviour may result

Environmental (social and physical) factors
Environmental factors may contribute to the problem of challenging behaviour where service users may react negatively to noise, heat and cold or to invasion of their personal space.
Some service users, particularly those with autistic spectrum disorders, may be over-sensitive to certain stimuli such as noise, echo, and may therefore react by displaying challenging behaviour.

Psychological trauma

- Reaction to abuse
- Bereavement – death of a loved

Medical factors

Medical factors include:

- pain or discomfort, illness or sensory difficulties;
- Some forms of challenging behaviour are particularly associated with certain conditions and disabilities such as repeated and involuntary body movements (tics) and uncontrollable vocal sounds (Tourette's syndrome) or ritualistic or obsessive behaviour (autistic spectrum disorders);
- Substance abuse – illegal drugs, alcohol etc.
- Neuropsychiatric disorders: epilepsy, Tourette's syndrome, attention-deficit hyperactivity disorder (ADHD);
- Syndrome-specific conditions and behavioural phenotypes such as Prader-Willi syndrome, Lesch-Nyhan syndrome, Williams syndrome.

Psychiatric factors

Psychiatric factors include:

- Depression.
- Mood disorders
- Schizophrenia

Warning signs of challenging behaviour

- increased restlessness;
- general body tension;

- irritation;
- withdrawal;
- refusal to communicate (refusal to verbalise their thoughts and feelings);
- general over-arousal of body systems (increased breathing and heart rate, muscle twitching etc.);
- pacing;
- increased volume of speech;

Types of challenging behaviour

- physical aggression – biting, hitting, kicking etc.
- violent behaviour;
- fire setting;
- inappropriate sexual behaviour – indecent exposure
- self-injurious behaviour (including ingestion or inhalation of foreign bodies);
- withdrawal and isolative behaviour;
- anger;
- self-neglect

Triggers of challenging behaviour

- Effecting change in repetitive and ritualistic behaviours, which are important ways of making the world safe to the individual.
- Effecting changes to routines without prior warning.
- Frustration when trying to communicate or not being allowed to speak out or get his /her point across.

- If the service user continues to see challenging behaviour as a means of problem-solving or gaining her/his objective.

- If the service user becomes bored and frustrated.

- If the service user perceives staff are not listening to him/her or not taking his/her unhappiness seriously.

- Strong expectations being placed upon a service user and lack of recognition at how well they are doing.

Guidelines for working with people with challenging behaviour

Care workers should at all times understand they have a legal duty to their safety first, their colleagues, people they support and visitors from their actions or omissions as outlined in Health and Safety at Work etc. 1974. Therefore, it is essential that all staff supporting someone with challenging behaviour should know:

- how to work safely and properly with the person taking into account:

o the person's communication potential/style;

o the person's patterns of communication – verbal, written, sign, symbols or objects; are you able to understand them?

o are the resources needed to achieve their understanding available? (Training, risk assessment, guidelines, etc.)

o is the person allowed to make informed choices?

o does the person have access to support and does he/she feel supported?

- Do you know the reporting procedures – recording information – how? by ticking charts, recording sheets and Antecedent – Behaviour – Consequences (ABC) charts

The role of the service manager

The service managers with the assistance from staff (regular/agency staff) should:

- carry out a risk assessment of each work situation, taking into account the individual being supported, the environment where the support is provided and furnishing that have the potential to be used as weapons on the care workers;

- take all necessary measures to eliminate risks found and where this is not achievable to reduce the risks to the lowest level practical as stipulated in the Health and Safety at Work Act 1974;

- ensure that all care workers who would be working with the individual have received appropriate training and are up to date with conflict management and physical intervention techniques;

- advise all employees of the risks to health and how these are to be avoided;

- in the circumstances where care workers raise a matter related to aggression and violence, steps should be taken to investigate the situation and take corrective measures where appropriate; this may mean revising the risk assessments and procedures;

- advise care workers of actions taken and records kept in regards to:

  o the risk assessments;

  o action taken as a result of the risk assessments;

  o information shared with care workers;

  o action taken in respect to incidents;

o   training – who has been trained and in what;

- have the behaviour support plan in place for all care workers working with service users with challenging behaviour that:

o   care workers will follow to provide individual support strategies aimed at reducing the incidence of challenging behaviour;

o   specifies the graded response needed to safeguard service users who challenge services through their behaviour;

o   describes individual primary and secondary prevention strategies and the safe and effective use of restrictive physical interventions;

o   describes the primary prevention strategies necessary to meet the complex support needs of service users with learning disabilities and autism that will prevent challenging behaviour;

o   describes the secondary preventions strategies that will distract or de-escalate a situation at an early stage that has the potential to escalate into an episode of challenging behaviour.

What you should do when challenging behaviour happens.

When faced with a challenging situation you should:

- appear calm and confident;
- be aware of a safe exit;
- speak clearly and calmly with a firm tone of voice;
- clearly state what is required;
- focus on behaviour, not the person;

27

- don't be challenging or aggressive;
- have confidence in your behaviour management skills;
- consider previous episodes of challenging behaviour;
- recognise positive behaviour and praise it;
- remain relaxed and breath normally;
- maintain comfortable eye contact but do not stare;
- keep movements slow and composed – quick actions may surprise and scare the other person.

Circumstances for using physical intervention

Physical intervention techniques are only for the use by trained staff when there is:

- significant risk of physical assault;
- a serious degree of urgency and danger;
- significant threats or attempts at self-injury;
- risk of serious accidents to self or others

Record all incidents and inform the manager and where necessary seek counselling to avoid psychological trauma.

Caution on Physical Restraint

The scale and nature of any physical intervention should be proportionate to both the behaviour of the individual to be restrained, and the nature of the harm they might cause either to themselves or to others.

The minimum necessary force should be used, and the techniques deployed should be those with which the staff involved are familiar with (trained) and able to use safely and are described in the service user's support plan

- all employees expected to work in areas that may require the restraint of violent or aggressive service users should have received training in the Management of Aggressive Behaviour including De-escalation Techniques and Peaceful Response Strategy

- Risk Assessments should be read, adhered to and used in conjunction with care plans with each service user

- Individual work places may have their own strategy on restraint and management of challenging behaviour and aggression and these should be adhered to. You should not get involved in service user restraint unless you have received appropriate training and have been deemed competent by the employer representatives (manager) to deal with situations requiring physical restraint.

- Physical restraint should always be a last resort. Only when all de-escalation techniques have failed, and where possible, the person in charge has given specific authority for an individual's involvement in restraint. Only safe and lawful techniques should be used.

- You are under no obligation to put your own personal safety at risk. If you are lone working, withdraw and seek help before the situation escalates.

- If supporting a service user where a clear risk of violence pre-exist, you should first seek full information and guidelines on the service user and support from the person in charge

- In the event of an injury, you should complete an incident form and the accident book and verbally report to the manager or person in charge.

CARE PROVISION

What is Social Care Provision?

Social care provision is the stipulation of personal care, social work, protection or social support services to adults and children in need or at risk or those who experience marginalisation or disadvantage or who have special needs

Understanding Care and its Delivery

Service users receive a comprehensive assessment of their needs and capabilities. They receive what is termed holistic assessment which means that they are viewed as a whole person who is living with learning disability. The assessment, therefore, considers physical, social, emotional, psychological and educational needs for each individual.

From this assessment a comprehensive plan of care is devised which involves a number of staff members providing different facets of care and a personalised, tailor-made care plan is formulated.

Care plan

What is a care plan?

A care plan is a structured, often multidisciplinary, task-oriented scheme, detailing the essential steps in the individual care of a service user and describing the likely course of their expected treatment and care. The care plan involves the translation of the needs, strength and risks identified into a written document that is responsive to the phase of the client's journey. The care plan should include:

- service user's name;
- key worker's name;
- identified goals in relation to specific support planned.

What is care planning?

Care planning is the process of setting goals and interventions based on the needs identified by an assessment and then planning how to meet those goals with the service user. Care planning is a core requirement of structured support

What is a service care plan?

The service care plan is devised when a service user moves into a care setting upon which support is made available and discussed and developed into an agreed service user care plan.

The care plan should include discussions and assessment of risks that the service user or staff may be exposed to as a result of the individual being able to make their own choices and decisions, which might result in conflict of interest in discharging duty of care, e.g. refusal to take prescribed medication by a service user.

A care plan should include:

- discussions and agreement of the service user, about who may be involved with the person's care needs;

- care planning and any required medications;

- therapies or interventions and any aims and goals to be achieved through the implementation of the individual's service care plan.

Assessment

The Support plan contains the service user's personal profile of their mobility status, moving and handling assessment, transfer procedures, medication administration, documentation (MAR Sheet) and storage. Staff should familiarise themselves with the care plans with the manager or supervisor to ensure they understand all that is required of them or any difficulties of which they should be aware.

Daily Activity Support Plan

The daily activity support plan should inform you what the service user needs, what and how these needs are to be met, from the service user waking up to getting dressed for the day. The personal care routine should spell out what support the service user needs and how often. For example showers on Monday, Wednesday and Saturday and a bath on Tuesday, Friday and Sunday

The personal care section should be as detailed as possible, for example, giving times of shower/bath if appropriate, equipment used and how to use it, routines the service user is familiar with and if any of the morning personal care routines need to be repeated throughout the day

The daily activity support plan should also include where the service user goes and at what time, equipment they might need, this should include any medication they need to take with them. It should also have instructions such as, whether you leave the service user with members of the support team e.g. at Day Centre, college or place of work. Transportation, what time they need to be picked up or dropped off back home etc.

The support you give the service user during activities should need also to be noted, giving as much details as possible. There should be separate instructions for meal times and medication routines (MAR Sheet should be followed).

All the above information should give you guidelines on what care the service user is receiving, instructions on what care you should deliver, how to move the service user and any identified hazards within the service user's living place.

Advocacy

Advocacy is defined as speaking up for, or pleading on behalf of another person or group. In practical terms this means ensuring that the service users are given information and the opportunity for input on any aspect of their own health care, and respect for their legal and moral rights

Service users may require an advocate for reasons such as;

- illness e.g. a stroke
- learning disability
- mental health problems
- limited knowledge, intimidation or embarrassment
- level of maturity
- where English is not their first language

In the course of your duty, if you believe a need for advocacy exists, discuss this with the manager who should determine what level of advocacy is required and should, if necessary, identify a competent third party or contact advocacy agencies.

General Duties of a Carer

The duties you are expected to perform for the service user although this is not a definitive list could include;

- o provide support with personal care i.e. washing/bathing, dressing and toileting
- o provide support that respects their dignity
- o assist them with administering, documentation and storage of medication
- o support with interacting with family and friends

o   assist with moving and handling (you should be trained and you are not expected to lift service users manually)

o   help maintain nutritional needs - that is; cooking meals, making drinks and assisting with feeding in accordance with dietary, religious or cultural requirements

o   assist with light household duties, dusting, hovering carpets, cleaning work surfaces and floors etc.

o   act as an advocate or support them to access advocacy agencies

o   promote and assist them to maintain independent living by engaging Active Support

o   other duties at the service user's or manager's discretion

Personal Care

Personal care includes: assistance with dressing, feeding, washing and toileting, as well as advice, encouragement, emotional and psychological support.

The Department of Work and Pensions (DWP) defines personal care as attention required in connection with bodily functions. These can include dressing, washing, bathing or shaving, toileting, getting in or out of bed, eating, drinking, taking medication, communicating etc.

Before commencing support with personal care ensure that you have the necessary equipment e.g. hoist and sling, gloves, razors etc.

Bathing, Showering and Washing of Vulnerable Individuals Safe Practice and Procedures

Bathing, showering and washing is a basic human need and care workers play a valued role in assisting people who are vulnerable because of their age, physical disability, mental health problems or a medical condition, particularly those that bring about sensory impairment.

When running a bath for a service user, run the cold water first, ensure that the bath water is not too hot before supporting a service user into the bath/shower. Take and record water temperature before immersing a person.

To prevent scalding the following precautions need to be in place and monitored by the manager or a team leader.

- A water thermometer needs to be available and used at all times before bathing starts.

- Notices should be placed in bathrooms instructing all care workers to check water temperatures before immersing a person in a bath tub

A water temperature log sheet should be filled in giving:

- water temperature

- date and time

- location – shower or bath

- service user's name

- name of the care worker and signature

Before assisting someone to a bathe you need to be informed and trained in the following;

- The use of special baths and any associated equipment such as hoists.

- Any special needs e.g. epilepsy or behavioural difficulties that the service user has

- To adhere to the relevant safety procedures, training and any instructions arising from the risk assessment.

In the event of an emergency pull the bath plug out and lift the individual's head clear from the water and call for help

If the hot water thermostat in a home is set too high record this on the log sheet and report it immediately to the manager.

Bathing/Showering

When undertaking personal care ensure you pay close attention to the following areas;

o **hair** – including scalp for soreness, dryness or flaky skin

o **skin** – check for breaks in the skin, cuts, bruises, infections, rashes or burns

o **mouth** – check that it is not dry, dentures are clean and fit well, teeth are brushed and mouth rinse used (where applicable) and that there are no sores on the tongue or inside of the mouth

o **Nails** – check the nails are clean, trim them if there is a care plan outlining this. Never cut a service user's nails especially if they suffer from diabetes.

o **Eyes** – check for stickiness of the eyelids, redness of the whites of the eye, any soreness or weeping.

o **Pressure Areas** – look for signs of pressure sores developing, sores/breaks in the skin. Check intact areas for blanching of the skin, the skin on pressure should turn from white to pink

As a care worker you are responsible for ensuring the water temperature is safe at all times, checking the temperature of water with a thermometer, and completing the log. Report any problems to the manager or supervisor immediately.

INCONTINENCE

What does incontinence mean?

Incontinence is the uncontrollable loss of urine or stool that is large or frequent enough to cause a social or health problem.

Incontinence can affect almost anyone during the course of their life and frequently occurs among the elderly and infirm service users. It is a problem that can be very upsetting and embarrassing. Your task is to support the service users to cope with the problem as well as possible with little disruption to their lifestyle. Always remember;

o   To preserve the service user's dignity

o   infection control measures - use of protective clothing, safe waste disposal, recognition of infection and hand washing

o   To apply the relevant aspect of your training e.g. the nature and effects of incontinence and its various types – loose stool or sign of constipation

o   To report any issues which arise in relation to a service user's incontinence to your manager or supervisor so that if necessary this can be taken further with their Healthcare professionals

Linen – contaminated (soiled) and clean linen should be kept separate. Place contaminated linen in a large **red** plastic bag and seal it before placing it in the washing machine. Remember to wash your hands

Always use a clean disposable sheet or incontinence pad when supporting a service user with incontinence. Change gloves after removing the contaminated pad before applying clean disposable pads. If in doubt contact your supervisor or manager

Privacy and Decency

When engaged in providing personal care, ensure that the service user's privacy is as great as the task permits, e.g. keep doors closed, keep them covered and ensure adequate but discreet supervision of the service user whilst he/she is bathing /showering and provide assistance as appropriate or as required

Always talk to the service user about their wishes in regard to dignity and privacy and observe these wishes.

Death of a Service User
If a service user is found dead in their own home or flat in case of shared accommodation, notify the service manager immediately for further instructions. Document any action taken in the service user's care plan.
In case of sudden death, call the paramedics, police and notify the service manager immediately; remain in the service user's home until the medical practitioner arrives.
o do not move, wash or otherwise disturb the body
o document any action taken in the service user's care plan
o return all completed service user's documentation to the service manager
o request for debriefing to avoid psychological trauma

HEALTH AND SAFETY
What is health and safety at work?

Health and safety at work is a government regulation that is used to protect the employee in a working environment. An employee has to enjoy the following rights; to have any risks to their health and safety properly controlled, to be provided, free of charge, with any personal protective and safety equipment

Employers Responsibilities

Section 2 *'Health and Safety at Work etc. Act 1974'* places a legal duty on the company to ensure so far as is reasonably practical, the health, safety, and welfare at work of all employees. It is the policy of the company to observe the requirements of the Health and Safety at Work etc. Act 1974 and any subsequent legislation or regulations and should include to;

- Provide health and safe systems of work, including a safe working environment, and premises with adequate amenities.
- Provide safe access and exit to and from the workplace.
- Ensure that you have appropriate training, instructions and supervision.
- Supply adequate information to employees so that they can ensure their own health and safety at work, and that of the people they work with.
- Have a written health and safety policy.
- Provide safe plants, machinery, equipment and appliances, and safe methods of handling, storing and transporting materials.

39

- Avoid hazardous manual handling operations, and where they cannot be avoided, reduce the risk of injury.
- Provide health surveillance as appropriate like CCTV to reduce the risk of damage, violence and disruption in the service.
- Ensure that appropriate safety signs are provided and maintained, e.g. exit signs on doors.

Your (employees) Responsibilities

Section 7 of Health and Safety at Work Act 1974, regulation 14 of the Management of Health and Safety at Work regulations 1999, as an employee you have legal duties and obligations to comply with individual duties. You have a duty to:

- take reasonable care of yourself and anyone else who might be affected by what you do at work or do not do;
- co-operate with the employer on health and safety matters;
- use correctly work items provided by the employer, including:
  o personal protective equipment, in accordance with training or instructions;
  o not interfering with or misuse anything provided for your health, safety or welfare at work.

Section 8 'Health and Safety at Work etc. Act 1974' states that "No person shall intentionally or recklessly interfere with or misuse any item provided in the interest of Health, Safety and Welfare"

Regulations 14 of the 'Management of Health and Safety at Work Regulations 1999', further extends their (employees) responsibilities:

"Every employee must use machines, equipment, dangerous substances, transport equipment, means of production or safety device provided by the employer, in accordance with the training and instructions received (whether this is written or verbal).

You should inform your employer of;

- any work situation where it is considered that the training and instructions received either directly by you or a colleague could represent a serious and imminent danger to their health and safety, and

- Any matter where it is considered that the training and instructions received by you or a colleague could present a failure in protection arrangements for their health and safety, even where no immediate danger exists.

It is a criminal offence for any employee to breach any of the aforementioned responsibilities.

National health and safety guidelines in the workplace

- All care workers and service users are obligated where appropriate to report hazards and to manage them in the first instance.

- All activities which are undertaken by staff should have been risk assessed and management controls should have been devised to manage them and all those taking part sign the risk assessment.

- Care workers who are working alone either in a project or in a client's home should follow the policies and procedures which detail what actions they should take to manage risks which may arise when lone working.

- To ensure a good standard of health and safety, and to maintain a good state of repairs by:

o Carrying out basic building checks and reporting any building defects;

o Fire checks on a weekly basis testing the fire alarms and smoke detectors to ensure they are in good working order.

- Every service should possess first-aid kits to manage minor injuries of self-injurious behaviour which the service users may present

Dealing with Emergencies in a Service User's Home

In general all care workers should know basic emergency first aid and when to call the emergency services. For instance when a service user have had an accident of;

- Small lacerations – clean with water or disinfectant and cover with a clean dressing
- Large lacerations – Call the emergency services. Cover with a clean dressing or tea towel; elevate the limb above the heart if possible to stop bleeding. If the bleeding does not stop apply pressure through the dressing or towel. Do not remove the towel/dressing to check if the wound has stopped bleeding, use another dressing or towel on top of the first ones.
- Small burns- Cool with cold water. If a blister appears do not burst it – cover with a dry dressing
- Large burns – call the ambulance. Lay the service user down and make them comfortable. Do not give them anything to eat or drink. Remain with the service user until help arrives.
- Water leaks – switch off the water from the stopcock and call the maintenance and inform the service manager
- Gas leaks – if you smell gas, open all doors and windows. Check that gas appliances are switched off. Turn off the gas mains and call the Emergency Gas Services immediately.

MEDICATION – ADMINISTRATION, STORAGE AND DOCUMENTATION

What is a medication?

A medication is a substance that is taken into or placed on the body that is used to cure a disease or condition, to treat a medical condition, to relieve symptoms of an illness or to prevent diseases.

Legislation requirements governing the management of medicines

There are two main statutes of law called 'Acts' from which regulations and orders arise that contribute to the regulations of medication within a care setting:

- The Medicines Act 1968
- The Misuse of Drugs Act 1971

The Medicines Act (1968) and the Misuse of Drugs Act (1971) dictates how medicines are managed and they should be complied with.

Drug classes

All drugs are given legal category to control how they are supplied to the public. The following abbreviations may be found on the packaging:

- POM   Prescription Only Medication
- P   Pharmacy Medicines: these medicines may only be sold in the pharmacy and the pharmacist should supervise the sale
- GSL   General Sales List: these medicines may only be sold in other stores such as supermarkets. Also known as household medicine

Occasionally you may come across other abbreviations either on the prescription or on the packaging. These are abbreviations for Latin words:

- TD   Twice Daily
- TDS   Three Times Daily
- QDS   Four Times Daily
- STAT   Immediately
- NOCTE   Night
- MAINE   Morning
- PRN   As and when required

Medication administration

When administering medication, you should know the therapeutic use of the medication administered, its normal dose, side effects, precautions and contra-indications of each drug. Before administering any prescribed drug, consult the person's medication administration sheet (MAR Sheet) and ascertain the following;

o Drugs – ensure that the service user is given the correct drug in the prescribed dose using the appropriate diluent (water, juice or food) and by the correct route

o Dosage - to protect the service user from harm, the dosage has been prescribed for the individual to ensure the effectiveness of the medication, taking into account height, weight, other medications being taken, severity of symptoms, likelihood and severity of side effects etc.

To administer medication follow this procedure:
- Select the service user's MAR sheet.

- Make sure the prescribed dose has not already been administered and note any changes in treatment (increase or decrease in dosage).

- Check that the prescription or the label on the medication is clear and unambiguous and relates to the service user in person.

- Check the identity of the service user (against the photograph on the medication folder).

- Administer the medication.

- Record on the MAR sheet immediately after the medicine has been taken.

- Record if the medicine is not taken, state the reason on the MAR sheet, the following letters should be entered in the box in place of a signature.

  A   refused

  B   nausea/vomit

  C   hospitalised

  D   social leave

  E   refused & destroyed

  F   other

  G   see note overleaf

- Where medicine is taken from the container and not taken by the service user, it should be stored in an envelope marked contaminated and returned to the dispensing chemist. It should never be replaced back in the container.

- Where the service user refuses to take their medicines, this should be reported to a senior member of staff or the manager who should then decide on what action to take or call NHS direct for advice. However, this is dependent on the nature of drugs prescribed.

Routes of administration

The route of medicines means the way in which medicines are taken or administered. The route and method of administration have been chosen for both its suitability to the individual and for the medication, to ensure it is absorbed in the most appropriate way. Route of administration is determined by its licence. The routes are;

- intra-aural – into the ears;

- inhalation – by nose or mouth into the lungs;

- intra-ocular – into the eyes;

- oral – by mouth;

- intramuscular – drug injected into the large muscle in the arm, leg or buttocks;

- intravenous – injected directly into a vein or cannula;

- rectal – introduced into the rectum through the anus;

- sublingual – under the tongue;

- topical – applied to the outer surface of the body, e.g. skin.

Procedure for the use of non-prescribed medication

- It is important to remember that you are not employed as a medical practitioner and should not therefore make decisions about medication people you are supporting require, without taking advice from a suitably qualified medical practitioner.

- All prescribed medication should be given exactly as instructed, unless advice has been sought from the person who prescribed it to adjust the time/dose as appropriate.

  Non-prescribed medication, such as simple cough linctus, should rarely be necessary as on most occasions someone who is unwell enough to need medication should be supported to see their GP.

  There are occasions when this is not necessary – for example with an occasional headache; on these occasions an over-the-counter remedy may be appropriate. However, medical advice should still be sought.

  This is to ensure that the proposed remedy:

- would not adversely affect prescribed medication already being taken;

- is appropriate for that particular individual and their medical history;

- is an appropriate treatment for the ailment causing discomfort.

  All medication should be booked in using the procedure in place even if that medication is a non-prescribed remedy.

As required ('PRN') medication

- 'As required' medication is prescribed by a General Practitioner or a healthcare specialist to treat various symptoms *occurring on an irregular basis.*

- These symptoms may include anxiety, maniac depression, tremors, and constipation among many others.

- Suggestions as to when it might be given should be supported by a care plan for you to follow.

- It is therefore important that the prescribed medication is offered at the appropriate time for each individual.

This should show:

o time of administration;

o dose given;

o initials of the care worker giving the medication

How medication arrives in the home/project

Medication is normally delivered to service users' homes in four different forms:

- Monitored Dosage System (MDS) (otherwise called a blister pack)

- Sealed packs - these are similar to the monitored dosage system but each pack contains only one tablet/capsule.

- Bottles for tablets/capsules or liquids - these are usually brown glass bottles with screw caps.

What are Controlled Drugs?

Some prescription medicines are controlled under the Misuse of Drugs legislation. These medicines are called controlled medicines or controlled drugs to prevent them:

- being misused, being obtained illegally or causing harm

Storage of Controlled Drugs (CD)

- Controlled drugs (CDs) are stored in a secure, cupboard that is used exclusively for CDs and those drugs that are managed in the same way.

- The cupboard which is often contained within a second cupboard is kept locked and access is restricted.

- The quantity and supply of these drugs is recorded in a Controlled Drug register. This book should be kept near the cupboard where the CDs are stored at all times and entries in it should be made, and checked by two staff, one of whom should be the shift leader whenever possible.

Medication best practice checklist

- Read the guidelines and always follow them.
- Always keep medicines in the same place in the cabinet.
- Keep bottles clean – wipe them if sticky or dirty.
- Lock the medication cabinet when not in use.
- Do not allow yourself to be distracted while you are in the process of administering medication.
- Never leave medication intended for one person, unattended in the presence of other service users

General information on medication

- Any increase or decrease in dosage should be authorised by a doctor. If this is done over the telephone, record the change and the name of the doctor in the service user's daily diary and notify all staff through the communication book.
- No one can be given medication prescribed for another service user except with the express authorisation of a doctor.
- Information on different medicines and their side effects can be found in the British National Formulary (BNF), a copy of which is kept in the offices of all care settings.
- If in doubt: ask, don't guess.

MOVING AND HANDLING

Definitions that apply to moving and handling:

- Any transporting or supporting of a load (including the lifting, putting down, pushing, pulling, carrying or moving thereof) by hand or by bodily force.
- Manual handling includes both transporting a load and supporting a load in a static posture. The load may be moved or supported by the hands or any other part of the body – for example, the shoulder.
- Manual handling also includes the intentional dropping of a load and the throwing of a load, whether into a receptacle or from one person to another. (The Manual Handling Operations Regulations)

You should have undertaken a Moving and Handling course before commencing duties that require Moving and Handling of service users. Ensure your Moving and handling certificate is up to date. (*We offer training. Email*

info@better-skills.co.uk)

It is imperative that you adhere to good safe working practices at all times.

- Under the legislation you as an employee are accountable for your own actions.
- Any lifting equipment or moving aids which have been supplied should be used in accordance with manufacturer's instructions.
- Do not make any repairs or carry out maintenance work of any description to moving and handling equipment.

The service users may be provided with equipment such as hoists, slings, sliding sheets, wheelchairs, bed pans, urinals,

50

foam cushions etc. Ensure you are aware of their correct usage.

Principles of Safe Handling

- Avoid lifting, use safe manual handling techniques or equipment where necessary

- Assess the task, service user/load, environment, equipment and your individual capability

- Plan the technique to be used and follow the instructions to be used. The moving and handling lead should give clear precise instructions (e.g. ready, steady lift)

- Explain to the service user what you are going to do and what s/he can expect

- Get help - Don't hesitate to ask questions or seek help if you are not sure of the procedure or your ability to handle the situation

Agency and bank staff

As an agency and bank care worker, you are regarded as employees for the purpose of compliance with arrangements for moving and handling. Employees have general health and safety duties to:

- adhere to and follow appropriate systems of work laid down for their safety;

- apply any manual handling training they have been given and comply with reasonable instructions on the performance of manual handling tasks;

- make proper use of equipment provided for their safety;

- cooperate with their employer on health and safety matters;

- inform the employer if they identify hazardous handling activities;
- take care to ensure that their activities do not put them or others at risk.

Moving and handling during emergency situations

In emergency situations, e.g. fire, it may be necessary to manually handle people to a place of safety as a matter of urgency. Employees should always use the best practical means of moving and handling without compromising the saving of life.

o Where a service user is observed to fall whilst you are present, you should first look after your own health, safety and welfare. You should refrain from the natural tendency to catch the service user to stop them from falling.

In such circumstances you should:

o allow the service user to fall naturally unless they are in danger, in which case, it would be appropriate to nudge them out of harm's way; or control the fall without taking all their weight, allow them to slide down your body, go with the service user to the floor, do not attempt to hold them up. Make them comfortable and call for help.

o ensure that the service user's head is protected from trauma, so far as is reasonably practicable.

Where a service user is discovered on the floor already, you should refrain from any attempt to immediately move them. In such circumstances, you should:

- examine the service user for injury and make them comfortable;
- assess the most appropriate means of moving the service user back to their bed or chair, this may include:

- advising the service user how to get up;

- using with colleague's assistance, an appropriate sling and hoist.

- If control and restraint are to be undertaken in an emergency situation, you should adhere to the techniques demonstrated in the control and restraint training programme and outlined in the care plan protocol

- Foreseeable emergencies should be assessed and have planned safe systems of work in place.

General information on manual handling

If you find a service user on the floor:

- do not attempt to lift him or her on your own;

- in the first instance check to see that they are 'safe';

- if they are unconscious, turn them into recovery position;

- summon assistance;

- if they are bleeding, it is stopped;

- no service user should be assisted off the floor;

- if the service user is conscious, ask if they are in pain;

- if the service user cannot get themselves up, you should call an ambulance, you should never lift them as they may have fractures.

FOOD HANDLING AND HYGIENE

What is food hygiene?

Food hygiene is a way of keeping food safe for consumption. In the case of care environment this means handling and keeping food safe for consumption by service users, residents and colleagues. The handling of food and food hygiene is regulated by the following legislation:

- Food Safety Act 1990: This legislation sets out the requirements of the food producer and handler with respect to food safety.

- Food Hygiene (England) Regulations 2006

Food Preparation

When preparing food the following are some of the guidelines to help ensure food safety:

- Observe good personal hygiene – wash hands regularly.

- Clean and sanitise equipment and surfaces thoroughly before and after use.

- Use different chopping boards/surfaces for raw food especially meat and ready to eat foods.

- Wash all fruits, vegetables and salads foods if being served raw.

- Keep all chilled foods and goods out of the fridge for the shortest time possible.

- Where possible use different equipment/utensils for raw foods and ready to eat foods.

- Avoid unnecessary handling of food.

- All foods should be used within three days of cooking, i.e. it is cooked one day, used the next day, and if not used all items should be thrown away on the third day

Food Handling

To ensure safe food handling, good hygiene practice should be followed at every stage, from receiving foods to serving of food by:

- keeping raw foods away from the ready-to-eat foods;
- storing dried foods off the floor, ideally in sealable containers, to protect from pests and contamination;
- never use food after the 'use by' date; make sure food rotation is practiced to ensure old supplies are used first
- observing temperature controls;
- following storage instructions on packaging and handling/labelling;
- checking deliveries are at the correct temperatures and that the food is not damaged (packaging/containers);
- using reputable suppliers whose supplies and sources can be easily traced back.

Food Storage

The temperature of all refrigerators should be:

- kept at 5 °C;
- freezers at -20 °C;
- checked twice daily by the staff on duty;
- recorded on the cold storage record sheet, dated and signed.

- All raw meats should be stored in a separate freezer or at the bottom of the refrigerator where it cannot come into contact with other foods.

- All foods should be covered and dated before being stored in the refrigerator. Especially leftovers (cooked) and dated when it should be used by.

Food can be contaminated by micro-organisms that multiply if the food is not stored correctly.

Food Preparation

- Care workers and service users engaged in the food handling process should at all times maintain the highest standards of personal hygiene and cleanliness consistent with Environmental Health recommendations.

- Care workers should encourage service users to assist in the kitchen subject to appropriate supervision and hygiene – washing hands before and after handling food.

- Any person working in the food area who knows or suspect that they are suffering from, or carriers of, any illness or condition likely to result in food contamination by micro pathogenis micro-organisms should advise the project or care setting manager as soon as possible.

- No persons who are known or suspected of suffering from, or the carrier of, any disease likely to be transmitted through food (e.g. by infected wounds and cuts, skin infections, diarrhoea or sores) should be allowed to work in any food handling area or cook for service users, if there is a possibility of contaminating the food

Causes of food poisoning outbreaks

Food poisoning is an acute illness usually occurring within 36 hours of consuming contaminated or poisonous food. Symptoms may last up to seven days and include:

- diarrhoea and vomiting

- fever and malaise

- abdominal pain and loss of appetite.

Food poisoning can be caused by:

- germs in food

- bacterial/toxins

- chemicals and metals in food

- viruses

- poisonous plants and fish.

Contamination can get into food in a number of ways:

- from raw (meat) food

- from dirty and contaminated work surfaces

- from pets and pest

- from packaging and equipment

- from cleaning products

- from you and your hands

  Safe food preparation, handling and storage in domestic and work environment will protect you and the service users from food poisoning.

INFECTION PREVENTION AND CONTROL

What is an infection?

An infection is the invasion of the body tissues by disease-causing organisms, e.g. bacteria or viruses; such micro-organisms are found in, around and on people and their surroundings at all times. (en.wikipedia.org/wiki/Infection)

Infection control is an issue of health and safety. It comes within the remit of Health and Safety at Work etc. Act 1974, Control of Substance Hazardous to Health Regulations 2002 and Personal Protective Equipment at Work Regulations 1992

Universal infection control precautions

The most important thing for a social care worker to do is to take steps to prevent infections by following the strict rules of universal infection control precautions. The term 'universal precautions' means undertaking safe working routine practices, to protect you and the service users from infection by blood and body fluids. Many diseases can be transmitted by infected blood or body fluids such as Hepatitis B, HIV and many others.

General safety on Infection Control

- Always cover any open wounds with a dressing or a waterproof plaster. Uncovered open wounds are subject to invasion by viruses, which could possibly enter into the bloodstream. All bodily fluids are potentially dangerous, especially when near open wounds.

- Always wear gloves and aprons when cleaning up spills from bodily fluids or excreta. Wash blood splashes off skin immediately with running water.

- Always wash your hands after you have finished each task and wash your hands before leaving the service user or finishing a specific care task.

- Never transfer the same pair of gloves from one service user to another: it may cause cross contamination. Use a new pair of gloves with each task.

- Cool burn injuries as quickly as possible by immersing the affected area in cold water or applying ice packs. Apply a sterile, dry dressing avoiding any constriction of the area. Do not apply any creams or ointments or lotions unless under medical advice. Do not prick any blisters.

- Always wear sensible shoes at work. Avoid wearing open footwear in settings where blood may be spilt, or where sharp instruments or needles are handled.

- Always wear sensible clothes at work.

- Remove all facial piercings whilst at work with the exception of small studs or similar and appropriate earrings to the ear lobe.

- There are lots of ways to ensure safety. Start by learning what hazards you may face for each part of your job. Then find out what steps you and the service users should take to stay safe and prevent accidents.

Sharps / Splash Injury

If you sustain a sharps or splash injury you should immediately;

- Encourage bleeding from the wound (sharp injury)

- The wound should be washed with warm running water and covered

- Skin, eyes or mouth (splash) should be washed with plenty of water
- The incident should be reported to the service manager and the accident book completed
- You should seek medical advice as soon as possible

HAND WASHING

When do you need to wash hands?

- Before starting work and after leaving the work area.
- Prior to serving meals and drinks
- Before and after each contact with the service users.
- After handling used laundry and clinical waste.
- After contact with bodily fluids.
- After removing disposable gloves.
- Before and after handling and eating food.
- After using the toilet.
- After touching or blowing your nose.

Body fluids procedures

Body fluid spills include blood, faeces, urine, vomit, tears, sweat, semen and anything else that comes from the person's body. Body fluid spills are a potential slip hazard. They may also potentially carry blood-borne viruses such as Hepatitis B & C and HIV, or other infections. Care must be taken when cleaning body fluid spills – always use a body fluid kit.

Body fluid Fit

The body fluid kit is labelled 'biohazard kit' and should be located in the main offices of the services or in COSSHI storage areas. The body fluid kit contains the following:

- a yellow coloured mop and bucket;
- disposable plastic aprons;
- disposable cloths;
- eye protectors;
- container of bactericidal cleaning liquid;
- disposable plastic gloves;
- yellow clinical waste sacks.

  NB: It is important to restock the kit after use and ensure that items remain in good condition.

Cleaning body fluid spills

Body fluid spill should be dealt with promptly. Where possible, the area should be blocked off and other people should be warned of the hazard to keep them away.

- Always wear plastic gloves and aprons and ensure that they are in good condition, i.e. gloves have no tears. Over boots (shoes protectors) and face mask should also be worn – personal protective equipment as stipulated in the Health and Safety at Work Act – The Personal Protective Equipment Regulations 1992. Failure to do so will be at staff members' own risk.

- Never reuse gloves or other personal protective equipment.

- Be aware that fluids may be present on other surfaces such as door handles, clothing, beddings and walls. Extra care should be taken if other objects such as sharps are also present.

- Always cover cuts and grazes with water proof dressings. Do not attempt to clear spills if you have eczema or chapped skin.

- Use bactericidal cleaning liquid by spraying on the spills and use paper towels to remove as much materials as possible. Spray the bactericidal liquid again and clean with hot water. Carpets should be shampooed where required.

- In order to avoid contaminating other surfaces when removing waste whilst wearing gloves, where necessary obtain help in opening doors.

- Dispose of all waste materials (other than sharps) and protective equipment in yellow clinical waste sacks and keep separate from other waste. Follow the procedures laid down by the organisation on clinical waste disposal.

Guidelines on Control of Substance Hazardous to Health (COSHH) and Personal Protective Equipment (PPE)

Under *COSHH or Control of Substance Hazardous to Health regulations 1994*, all persons need to know the safety precautions to take so as not to endanger themselves or others through exposure to substance hazardous to health.

There are four general classification of risk;

- Toxic – may cause death or acute or chronic damage to health when inhaled, swallowed or absorbed via the skin

- Corrosive – may on contact with living tissues, destroy them

- o Harmful – may cause death or acute chronic damage to health when swallowed or inhaled

- o Irritant – may cause inflammation

  For safety precautions;

- You should be provided with gloves, aprons and shoes protectors for handling body or clinical waste in accordance with the PPE 1992 regulations

- Store all chemicals and cleaning materials in a safe secured place out of reach of service users or children

- Never mix cleaning chemicals or transfer them into another container.

- When using bleach or cleaning fluids always wear gloves

- Splashing of eye with any product should be followed immediately by rinsing with clean, running cold water for 5 – 10 minutes and medical attention should be sought immediately

  Any accident or incident to yourself or the service user should be reported to the service manager or supervisor and recorded in the Accident Book and medical advice sought

FIRE SAFETY

What are fire prevention measures?

Fire prevention measures refer to precautions that are taken to prevent or reduce the likelihood of a fire that may result in death, injury, or property damage. The measures that should be taken include;

Risk assessment

Assessments should include:

- identifying hazards and people at risk including those with disabilities;

- removing or reducing the hazards and managing the remaining risks to acceptable levels;

- contacting your local fire service to visit and give safety advice and talk to both the care workers and service users.

Safety

- The manager or team leader should act as the fire warden for the project/residential setting and be responsible for the evacuation of the premises in the event of fire and fire drills.

- The manager should ensure that regular fire alarms and smoke detectors tests take place (weekly), escape lighting checks (monthly) and evacuation drills (quarterly) are carried out and records kept.

Training/awareness

- The project/residential managers should ensure that all staff are, and remain, familiar with the relevant fire and emergency procedures for the project/residential/supported living schemes/care setting.

- Managers should also arrange for staff training that may be appropriate (e.g. using fire blanket, what type of fire extinguishers to be used on what types of fire, i.e. electricity, gas, wood etc.).

Some of the causes of fire in the home are;

- Faulty electrics – electrical appliances
- Open fires – wood- burning stoves
- Candles and Cigarettes
- Furnaces, Fireplaces, and Electrical Heaters
- Chips pan fires

Electrical Equipment

- Always use an electrical circuit breaker (residual current device – RCD) with any appliance – such as vacuum cleaner, electrical kettle etc.
- Check for signs of loose wiring and faulty plugs and sockets.
- Replace any worn or taped-up cables and leads.
- Don't overload sockets.
- Don't put cables under carpets or mats.
- Check the maximum amps that the fuse in a plug can handle.
- Turn off equipment and unplug it when not in use. Store it in a safe place.
- If you need to use an adapter, ensure it has a fuse and keep the total output to no more than 13 amps.

Do not touch anyone who have been electrocuted until you have isolated the electricity supply (turn off at the mains) call the emergency services

Be prepared in event of fire

Everybody affected should be aware of what to do and how to escape in the event of fire.

- Escape routes should be planned and exits kept clear. Keep doors and window keys handy, where applicable.

- Ensure fire safety risk assessment is conducted and reviewed at least annually or when need arises.

- Ensure that regular fire alarms tests are carried out weekly, emergency lighting checks monthly and evacuation drills are carried out quarterly.

- Make sure all relevant fire exit and evacuation signs are in place.

- Test smoke alarm batteries regularly (where applicable).

- Consider how anyone with restricted mobility (e.g. a wheelchair user) or other disability would evacuate the building.

- If a fire starts and there is smoke, keep low where the air is clearer.

- Keep fire doors closed to prevent fire from spreading.

Evacuation - Know how to respond in the event of a fire

- Stay calm – and help service users to stay calm.

- Help service users leave the building using the nearest exit.

- Alert everyone in the house by shouting fire or breaking the fire glass panels to sound the alarm.

- Contact the fire brigade from a neighbour's house or a mobile phone.

- Keep a head count for all service users and staff.

- If you are unable to remove a service user, keep the fire door shut and get help as soon as possible – do not put yourself at risk.

If the escape route is blocked

- You may be able to escape from a window if you are on ground or first floor – only consider this option as a last resort.

- Don't jump. Lower yourself from the ledge before dropping – this should break your fall.

- Where possible throw beddings, cushions etc. outside to break your fall.

- Shut the doors and use beddings and clothes to block the bottom of the door, this should prevent smoke from entering the room if it's not a fire door.

- If you can't escape from the building through windows get everyone into one room (probably with a telephone and a window).

- Shout for help from the window if necessary.

- Avoid opening the fire doors as they are meant to keep smoke out and air (wind) which help accelerate the fire.

- Lean out of the window to breathe if you have to from time to time.

If your clothes catch fire

- Don't run around – this will only fuel the flames.

- Lie down and roll – it smothers the flames, which makes it harder for the fire to spread and helps protect your face and (head) hair - flames burn upwards.

- Smother the flames by covering them with heavy material like a coat or blanket.

- Remember the basic principles when on fire – stop! drop! and roll!

Types of Fire Extinguisher for Homes

Water Fire Extinguishers - good for tackling fires involving burning paper, wood and soft furnishing (Class A fires)

Foam Fire Extinguishers, also called AFFF FOAM (Aqueous Film Forming Foam) - create a smothering film of foam over the fire, which starves the fire of oxygen.

CO2 (Carbon Dioxide) Fire Extinguishers contain only pressurised CO2 gas. Good for burning liquids (Class B fires), and electrical fires.

Powder Fire Extinguishers, such as ABC powder extinguishers or dry powder extinguishers, are suitable for fighting class A, B and C fires.

Wet Chemical Fire Extinguishers are especially designed for use on kitchen fires involving burning oil and deep fat fryers (Class F fires).

NB: Don't attempt to use an extinguisher on a fire unless you feel it is safe for you to do so.

Fire blanket - designed to extinguish small incipient (starting) fires especially in the kitchen.

EQUALITY, DIVERSITY AND DISCRIMINATION

What is equality?

Equality is ensuring individuals or groups of individuals are treated fairly and equally and no less favourably, specific to their needs, including areas of race, gender, disability, religion or belief, sexual orientation and age.

Equality (equal opportunities)

Equal opportunities are about providing fair and equal access/treatment for everybody regardless of their age, race, gender, disability, religion or belief and sexual orientation

What is diversity?

Diversity is about creating a working culture that seeks to respect value and harness differences, rather than judging people and ideas by the extent to which they conform to our existing values, recognising that those differences provide opportunities for a richer, more creative business environment that can better provide for the diverse nature of everyone.

Diversity is proactive and inclusive, taking in visible differences such as gender, ethnicity and disability, as well as differences that are not necessarily and immediately apparent, such as sexual orientation, religious beliefs and nationality.

Factors that may lead to social exclusion

Social exclusion means that service users are excluded from joining society through 'factors beyond their control'. These might be issue such as:

- insecure, low paid, low quality employment;

- low levels of education, illiteracy;

- growing up in a vulnerable family (e.g. single parent, domestic violence);

- disability;

- poor health; physical or mental health problems

- living in a multiple deprivation (crime, drugs, antisocial behaviour);

- homelessness and precarious conditions;

- immigration, ethnicity, racism and discrimination;

- de-institutionalisation (prisons, institutional care, mental institutions);

- age

The Nine Strands of Diversity (protected characteristics)

There are Nine Strands (protected characteristics) of diversity, which cannot be used as a reason to treat people unfairly. Every person has one or more of the protected characteristics; The Equality Act 2010 that came into effect in October 2010 protects everyone against unfair treatment.

The Nine strands of Diversity include;

- Age
- Disability -
- Gender
- Marriage and civil partnership
- Pregnancy and maternity

- Race and ethnicity
- Religion and belief
- Sexual orientation
- Transgender

Cross Gender Care

Service users should feel free to decide the gender of their care workers and these issues should be agreed at the commencement of care. "Same gender is not mandatory, however, cultural and religious needs should be taken into account.

Supporting service users in upholding their rights

You can help service users in upholding their rights by:

- listening – using your communication skills to accurately find out their needs;
- always ensuring that their needs are met promptly and in full;
- maintaining a pleasant attitude;
- ensuring that your communication is open and honest;
- developing a professional relationship;
- ensuring you work within the service user's care plans;
- referring to legislation, codes of practice, policies and procedures to guide you in your practice;
- giving people information that they need – it is essential that this information is relevant, up to date and provided in a way that is appropriate to the service user – e.g. speech/vocalisation, signing, the use of Makaton,

symbols/objects of reference for some service users with learning disabilities, and translating information into community languages or large prints, or Braille form.

Anti-discriminatory practice

Promoting equality, diversity and rights

- When working with people with learning disabilities, it is essential that we consider the way in which we think about and treat them.
- Service users should be worked with in a way that demonstrates we accept them as individuals by respecting and valuing them and treating them equally.
- This is in recognition that service users have particular rights in the care they receive.
- Staff need to be aware of the rights of service users and be able to distinguish these from responsibilities.
- You should examine ways to ensure that service users have access to their rights.

Legislations

The laws relating to rights and equality that are most relevant to care and those that you need to have a basic understanding of are summarised below.

- Care Standards Act 2000
- Disability Discrimination Act 2005
- Equality Act 2010
- NHS and Community Care Act 1990
- The Children's Act 1989
- The Data Protection Legislation 1998

ABUSE – SAFE GUARDING OF VULNERABLE ADULTS

Definition of abuse

Abuse is a violation of an individual's human and civil rights by any other person or persons. (Department of Health, 2000)

Why does abuse happen?

Abuse happens due to one or a combination of the above factors;

- Inadequate training of carers.
- Lack of person-centred care planning or a ritualised care routine.
- Working in isolation.
- Continued over-demanding behaviour (challenging behaviour)
- Communication difficulties.
- Drug and alcohol abuse.
- Stress within a relationship.
- Lack of support and or services.
- Reversal of roles – abused becomes the abuser.
- Poorly supervised carers/services

Types of Abuse

Physical abuse

Physical abuse is one of the most common types of abuse. It can take place in many ways: hitting, slapping, rough handling, inappropriate restraints or sanctions, excessive or inappropriate use of medication.

Indicators of physical abuse can be in form of physical or behavioural indicators.

1. *Physical indicators*

(a) Unexplained bruises, welts, lacerations and abrasions:

- on the face, lips, mouth;
- on torso, back, buttocks, thighs;
- lacerations in various stages of healing;
- reflecting shape of an article used, e.g. belt buckle;
- bite marks or fingernail marks, scratches.

(b) Unexplained burns:

- especially on soles, buttocks, arms, or back;
- immersion burns;
- electric burns (iron);
- rope burns.

(c) Unexplained fractures

- to the skull, facial structure;
- fractures in various stages of healing;
- multiple or spiral fractures.

2. *Behavioural indicators*

- reluctant to change clothes in front of others.
- wary of adult contact.
- difficult to contact.

- Apprehensive when children cry.

- Crying/irritability.

- Frightened of formal and informal carers.

- Behavioural extremes – aggression, withdrawal, impulsiveness.

- Apathy.

- Depression.

- Poor peer relationships.

- Panic in response to pain.

Neglect

Neglect occurs when a service user is not provided with adequate care and attention and suffers harm or distress as a result. Neglect and acts of omission include ignoring medical or physical care needs; failure to provide access to appropriate health, social care or educational services; the withholding of the necessities of life, such as medication, food, drink and heating.

Indicators of neglect

1. Physical indicators

- constant hunger;

- failure to thrive or malnutrition;

- poor hygiene which may result in health problems;

- unattended physical problems or medical needs.

2. *Behavioural indicators*

- stealing food;

- constant fatigue, listlessness or falling asleep;

75

- alcohol or drug abuse;
- aggressive or inappropriate behaviour;
- isolation from peer group.

Emotional/psychological abuse

This can be more difficult to define and measure, because of this, it is often more difficult to detect and identify. Most obviously it can be seen as cruelty or verbal insults, but it can include shouting and swearing at service users, or even spreading rumours, malicious gossip or withholding of duty of care.

Indicators of emotional/psychological abuse

- Extreme low self-esteem.
- Compliant, passive, withdrawn, tearful, aggressive or demanding behaviour.
- Depression.
- Constant high anxiety.
- Poor social and interpersonal skills.
- Delayed development, i.e. speech.
- Persistent habit disorder, e.g. rocking, biting.
- Self-destructive behaviour.

Sexual abuse

Sexual abuse is any contact or interaction (physical, visual, verbal or psychological) between a child/adolescent and an adult (or another adult) when the child/adolescent/adult is being used for the sexual stimulation of the perpetrator or any other person, and – in the case of adults – without the mutual consent of both parties.

- Sexual abuse in the care setting is where the service user is forced to take part in sexual activity without their consent.

- Any kind of sexual relationship between a staff member and a service user is abusive, even if consent is given.

- However, sexual abuse can take more subtle ways and can occur when staff are administering personal care, or making comments related to someone's sexual orientation or gender identity.

Indicators of sexual abuse

- Unexplained difficulty walking.

- Bleeding or bruised genitals.

- Complaining of pain while urinating or having a bowel movement, or exhibiting symptoms of genital infections such as offensive odours, or symptoms of a sexually transmitted disease.

- Reluctant to be alone with a particular person.

- Sudden behaviour change.

- Engaging in persistent sexual play with friends, toys or pets.

- Having unexplained periods of panic, which may be flashbacks from the abuse.

- Regressing to behaviours too young for the stage of development they already achieved.

- Initiating sophisticated sexual behaviours.

Institutional abuse

Institutional abuse is the mistreatment of people brought about by poor or inadequate care or support or systematic poor practice that affects the whole care setting. It occurs when the individual's wishes and needs are sacrificed for the smooth running of a group, service or organisation.

This type of abuse can be rife in areas where there is a very rigid and long-standing routine ('we have always done it that way.') Or when tasks are carried out for the 'good' of the staff, rather than in the best interest of service users, e.g. bath times, weigh days in prison or residential homes.

Indicators of institutional abuse

- Treating adults like children.

- Arbitrary decision making by staff group, service or organisation.

- Strict, regimented or inflexible routines or schedules for daily activities such as meal times, bed/waking times, bathing/washing, going to the toilet.

- Lack of choice or options such as food and drink, dress, possessions, daily activities and social activities.

- Lack of privacy, dignity, choice or respect for people as individuals.

- Unsafe or unhygienic environment.

- Lack of provision for dress, diet or religious observance in accordance with an individual's belief or cultural background.

- Withdrawing people from individually valued community or family contact.

Financial abuse

Financial abuse can take many forms, from staff denying service user all access to funds, to making them solely responsible for all finances while handling money irresponsibly themselves. Or this is the attaining of money, possessions or property through cheating or deception.

Indicators of financial abuse

- Sudden withdrawal of money from bank accounts.

- Loss of financial documents.

- Person with a disability is accompanied by family, care worker or others who appear to coax, or otherwise pressure, the individual into making transactions.

- Persons accompanying the individual speak for her/him, and do not allow the individual to speak or make decisions.

- Individual expresses concern that s/he does not have enough money for basic needs.

- Individual is confused about missing funds in accounts.

- Sudden increase in checking overdrafts.

- Unusually large cash withdrawals or transfers to other accounts from a joint bank account, without the individual's knowledge or consent.

- Individual cannot obtain checking or savings passbooks from person assisting with finances, or passbook/cheque book are frequently missing.

- Individual complains that furniture, jewellery, credit cards, or other items are missing.

- The individual complains about not having access to her/his own money.

- Caregiver charging personal expenses to the credit card of an individual or using the service users monies for personal groceries

Discriminatory Abuse

Discriminatory abuse occurs when values, beliefs or culture result in a misuse of power that denies mainstream opportunities to some groups or individuals.

It is the exploitation of a person's vulnerability, which excludes them from opportunities in society. This could include;

- unequal treatment due to race, gender, religion, age, sexuality or disability

- verbal abuse, inappropriate language, slurs, harassment and deliberate exclusion

- denial of basic human and civil rights e.g. allowing people to follow their own spiritual or cultural beliefs or choice about their own sexuality

- failure to meet and take into account religious and cultural needs of an individual

- racist graffiti or bringing racist material (magazines, leaflets) into the vulnerable individuals home.

Indicators of discriminatory abuse may include:

- lack of choice

- lack of privacy and dignity

- lack of personal belongings

- use of punishment - withholding food and drink

- tendency for withdrawal and isolation

- expression of anger or frustration or fear and anxiety

- lack of disabled access

- being refused access to services or being excluded inappropriately.

  The indicators of discriminatory abuse may take the form of any of the other types of abuse. The difference lies in that the abuse is motivated by discriminatory attitudes, feelings or behaviour towards an individual or a group.

What can you do to stop abuse?

- You should always act.
- Know the organisation's procedure for reporting abuse.
- If you suspect abuse, inform the line manager immediately.
- Speak to a service user's social worker.
- In the event of criminal behaviour, inform the police.
- Always check that action has been taken.
- Do not try too much by yourself.
- Respect the wishes of the individual and be sensitive to their cultural background.
- Do not promise to keep secrets.
- If possible act with the knowledge of the service user. If this is not possible you should still take action.
- Be aware of the need to protect and not contaminate evidence.
- Information that should be required should include what you have been told, by whom, what you yourself have observed, dates, times, locations, names, etc. Do not embroider the facts.
- Document and record everything.

Strategies to Prevent Abuse

To be able to prevent abuse there are certain things we should consider before every contact, intervention or response with the service user. We should always ask ourselves 'Is this in the best interest of the service user?' Every care worker should be able to justify their answer to this question.

There are five levels which we have to be aware of to be able to prevent abuse:

a) Service user

b) Yourself (care workers, volunteers, caregivers etc.);

c) Environment;

d) Organisation;

e) Current legislation and guidance.

(a) Service user

In order to prevent a potentially abusive situation from arising in a care environment you should consider the following about the service user:

- Is there a care plan in place?

- Do you know it?

- What is the service user's wishes and preference?

- What is the communication potential/style? Verbal or nonverbal?

- What is the service user's pattern of communication – oral, written, sign, symbols or objects? Are you able to understand them?

- Are behaviour support plans in place?

- What is the mental/physical state of the service user?

- What control measures are in place?

- Has intervention been risk assessed?

- What has worked before?

- Can you avoid the intervention?

- Have other tactics be tried such as de-escalation?

(b) Yourself (care worker, volunteers etc.)

As a member of the care team, consider how you could prevent a potentially abusive situation from arising by bearing in mind the following;

- Do you know the organisation's policy and procedure on safeguarding?

- Do you know the care plan? Has it changed recently?

- Do you know the potential risks involved, and how you can avoid them?

- Are you trained to do this?

- Do you know how to access support?

(c) Environment

With the insight knowledge you have on the service user, you should assess how you could contribute towards preventing abuse from arising by considering the following in regard to environment:

- Is the area safe for the service user, is it too hot/cold/noisy? Are lights too dim/bright etc.?

- Are there any trip hazards, sharps, electricity, etc.?

- Are there doors/windows; are these closed, in the toilets and bathrooms?

- Are doors locked? Can they ensure privacy and dignity?

(d) Organisation

As care worker, you should be able to know what the management can do to help combat the threat of abuse. The management should ensure that the potential for abuse is recognised and that strategies are put in place by:

- ensuring care plans are in place;

- the risk assessments are carried out, reviewed and up-to-date;

- training is up-to-date; who is trained in what;

- running Criminal Records Bureau checks;

- the staffing level is adequate;

- ensure consent is obtained on issues of confidentiality where appropriate;

- the care setting is registered with the relevant body (usually Care Quality Commission – CQC).

(e) Current Legislation and Guidance

The organisation does not expect the care workers to know the content of all pieces of legislation; however, you are expected to familiarise yourself with them, know and work within the organisation's policies and procedures that relate to your work.

The following legislation or guidance should be available in place to raise awareness to avoid abuse. Depending upon the area, the legislation and guidance include:

- The Children and Young Persons Act 2008

- Deprivation of Liberty Safeguards Act 2007

- Mental Health Act 2007

- Safeguarding Vulnerable Groups Act 2006

- The Care Standards Act 2000

- NHS & Community Care Act 1990

- Offences Against the Person Act 1861

- Domestic Violence and Matrimonial Proceedings Act 1976

- Race Relations Act 1976

- The Human Rights Act 1998

- Sexual Offences Act 2003

- The Disability Discrimination Act 2005

Ways to prevent abuse

There are different ways that can help stop or prevent abuse from occurring in any care environment. Prevention needs to take place in the context of person-centred support and personalisation, with individuals empowered to make choices and supported to manage risks.

- The most common prevention intervention for adults at risk include training and education of the adults at risks themselves and staff on abuse in order to help them to recognise and respond to abuse.

- Other approaches include identifying people at risk of abuse.

- Raising awareness, information, advice and advocacy, policies and procedures, community links, legislation and regulations, interagency collaboration and a general emphasis on promoting empowerment and choice.

- Education: this involves providing service users with knowledge about their rights, and teaching them skills to identify abuse, ask for help, and avoid being re-victimised.

- Care workers and caregivers need information and support to help them care for service users in a positive and an empowering manner.

- Increase knowledge about service users' abuse and its impact throughout different stages of life.

Organisations involved in safeguarding (prevention of abuse)

There are some key organisations/agencies that may need to be involved in safeguarding concerns (abuse). It should be the service manager or senior staff in the management who should decide who to contact and take action in doing so, or you should know the procedure to follow. Below are some of those to contact.

Police

Care workers in a care environment should know the procedures of contacting the police, if at any time the situation involves something which is against the law or the service user or a witness is in danger, the police should be contacted immediately or at the earliest opportunity. The person in charge of the service should initiate this contact. In such cases, the police will need to gather evidence.

Local Authorities Designated Officer (LADO)

All care workers and volunteers should know that each local authority has a LADO who should be alerted to all cases in which it is alleged that a care worker or volunteer who works with vulnerable people has behaved in a way that has harmed or may have harmed a vulnerable person, or has committed a criminal offence against a vulnerable

person or their behaviour towards vulnerable people
indicates she/he is unsuitable to work with vulnerable
people.

Social care team

The local authority social care team should be notified of
any safeguarding concerns about any vulnerable person/
child, and if the vulnerable person/child has a social
worker, they should be contacted. In cases of registered
looked after children, the concerned teams should be
contacted as well.

Adult social care team

If the vulnerable person is an adult, the local social services
office or the named care manager should be notified. Each
and every vulnerable adult in any setting has a care
manager who oversees their well-being; from housing
needs, benefits etc. the local authority safeguarding team
will consider the referrals, and offer advice on what action
should be taken in response.

Recording observable body injuries

The physical injuries or unexplained bruises found on the
body of a service user should be shade and labelled on a
diagram called a 'body map', the size, shape and colouring
should equally be noted, this may help determine when the
injuries occurred. Fill an incident/accident form and police
reference numbers or any other authority that may have
been contacted.

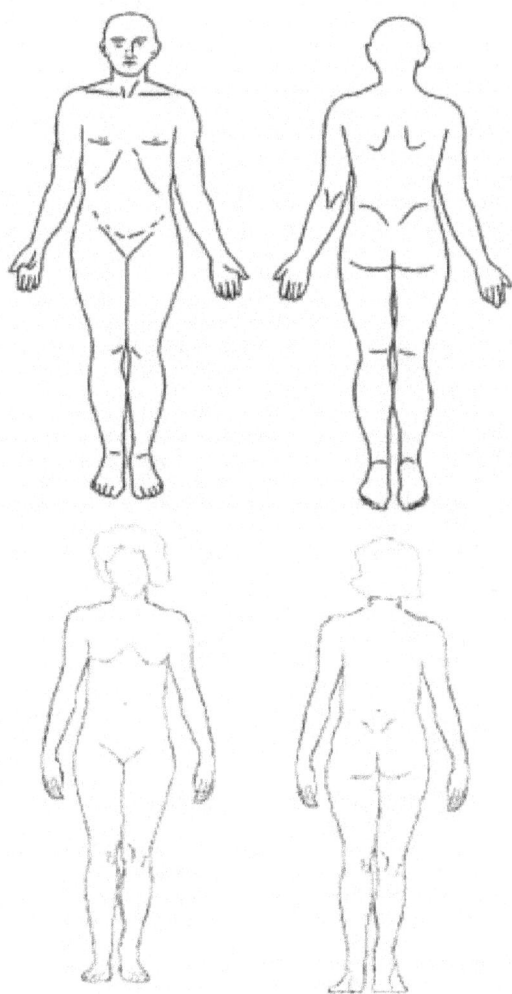

Body Map

LONE WORKING

Who is a lone worker and what is lone working?

Lone workers are defined by Health and Safety Executive as 'those people who work by themselves without close or direct supervision'. This may include those who work alone in specific areas or buildings such as supported living schemes, hostel, housing projects workers, key workers, single cover scheme workers, community floating support, tradespersons to name a few.

Lone working is covered by the Health and Safety at Work Act 1999 and the Management of Health and Safety at Work Regulations 1974. This legislation applies to all instances of lone working. Many organisations use the term 'lone worker' to describe an employee who normally works alone in a service or someone who provides support to clients in their own homes. They may be part of a team, but work on their own routinely and are not closely supervised. They may be office-based employees, Floating support workers working in the community. They may be permanent or agency employees in a service.

Guidelines on Lone Working

- All lone workers should be inducted thoroughly and receive a full handover before commencing their duties.

- They should be given information to deal with normal everyday situations but should also understand when and where to seek guidance from others in unusual or threatening situations like calling the police.

- All lone workers should have had a full Criminal Records Bureau check before commencing lone working for any care setting.

- All lone workers should read, sign and understand the professional boundaries and protection from abuse policies. This knowledge should be updated regularly.

In accordance with these policies of professional boundaries:

o lone workers are not permitted to act inappropriately towards the service users;

o lone workers should not make physical contact with the service users unless it is documented in their plan of care and this is also dependent on the nature of services provided

o lone workers should not say anything inappropriate to any service users at any time.

As a lone worker you should have regular reviews with the line manager in the workplace to ensure your knowledge of lone working policy is up to date and appropriate for continued lone working.

As a lone worker, you should at all times carry a portable (mobile) phone, whether one provided by the project or your own. (In most cases, projects/homes provide a mobile phone as additional equipment for safety.)

Possible risks faced by a lone (care) worker in a service user's home

Lone working is seen as the most appropriate and positive way of offering support to service users. However, there is some possible risk a care worker could face:

- verbal/physical attack resulting in psychological harm
- a lone worker could be verbally or physically attacked; for instance if the service user is under the influence of alcohol

or they are distressed or angry to the point where they lash out blindly;

- a care worker could have allergic reaction to pets;

- a care worker could be bitten by a dog or scratched by a cat or a hamster;

- Unpredictable and possible violent reactions towards a care worker causing psychological or physical harm, especially when a task is likely to generate a hostile reaction from the service user.

Lone working in a service user's home

Responsibility of employers

According to Health and Safety Executive, employers of lone workers should:

- involve staff or their representatives when undertaking the required risk assessment process;

- take steps to check control measures are in place (examples of control measures include instructions, training, supervision and issuing protective equipment);

- review risk assessment annually or, as few workplaces stay the same, when there has been a significant change in working practice; when a risk assessment shows it is not possible for the work to be conducted safely by a lone worker, risks should be addressed by making arrangements to provide help or back-up;

- where a lone worker is working at another employer's workplace, that employer should inform the lone worker's employer (recruiting agency) of any risks and the required control measures.

Responsibility of staff

- Staff to respect the personal space of the service user they visit in their own homes.

- To take a flexible and responsive approach to the individual needs and wishes of each service user.

- To identify and promote best practice in supporting service user to enhance safe lone working.

  When working in a service user's home, it is important to remember that staff are visitors and that they are entering the service user's private space and it should be respected as such.

Good Principles for lone working in service user's home

1. Acceptable behaviour from a lone worker

- Calling before going over to announce your arrival time if it is not a shift working pattern.

- Knocking on the door and waiting to be invited in.

- Showing your identification and stating your business, e.g. link work.

- Asking to use facilities in the house such as:

o the toilet;

o kettle and beverages to make a cup of tea/coffee;

o to change Television channels

o to open the windows and curtains: for some service users it's part of their morning routine/ritual and should be considered as a possible trigger for anxiety or challenging behaviour. There are usually guidelines in regards to this.

2. Behaviour unacceptable from a lone worker

- Knocking on the door and walking in without being invited in.

- Not acknowledging the service user as you walk into the house without greetings.

- Walking into the kitchen and helping yourself to tea/coffee without asking.

- Opening windows and curtains without asking.

- Using bathroom without asking.

- Not introducing yourself to the service user.

  At the same time, when you are working in a service user's home, it is your workplace and you remain responsible for your own health and safety. It is important, therefore, to maintain and reflect professional values and principles regarding working effectively with service users at all times.

When leaving the house in case it is not a 24 hours care;

- Check that the service user is comfortable and that everything necessary is within easy reach.

- Check that potential sources of danger are not accessible, particularly if the service user has any disability e.g. visual impairment

- make sure that appliances which are no longer needed are switched off

- Make sure that the home is secure. If leaving during the day, ensure that the service user knows which windows are open, if any and are easily accessible for them to close.

Lone working in an emergency situation

- If lone working in the community you should try to get to a place of safety walking along places with CCTV, or at least a public place. Then you should use the mobile phone to call the project or the police if necessary.

- If you feel at risk, and cannot get to a safe place or a public place, you should call the project and inform them where you are using the password or the sentence or code for emergency. This should alert your colleagues that you feel you are in danger and the colleagues should act upon your message and call 999, alert the police as to where you are and other details of the situation that they know.

- If lone working on the project with another member of staff in a different area of the project, return to the office and lock the door if it's safe to do so and if possible call the other member of staff to return to the office and if necessary call the police to attend if you feel unsafe.

Emergency recovery plan when lone working

Every organisation should have their own emergency procedures in place, which describe what to do in the event that someone does not check in or calls for help in an emergency or in event of a crisis. If a lone worker has not checked in or come back at the time they had stated:

- The first thing to do is call the mobile phone number they are carrying, and if there is no response call their personal mobile phone and leave a message, as they may just have forgotten to check in.

- Wait for a certain length of time – this should be dependent upon agreement of what is appropriate for different situations. In some circumstances staff should not wait at all but proceed straight away to emergency procedures.

- If there is no response, staff should advise the project manager or other colleagues.

- Establish their last expected location and if possible try to contact that place.

- If concern is high, police should be contacted and arrange an immediate police visit to their last known location.

VIOLENCE AT WORK

Definitions of violence

The Department of Health has defined violence and aggression as 'any incident where staff are abused, threatened or assaulted in circumstances relating to their work, involving an explicit or implicit challenge to their safety, well-being or health'.

In accordance with the Health and Safety Executive, violence at work is defined as 'any incident in which a person is abused, threatened or assaulted in circumstances relating to their work'. Abuse on the other hand includes verbal abuse in all degrees or threats and counts just as much as a physical attack.

Types of violence at work

- shouting verbal/racial/sexual abuse
- pushing
- spitting
- objects thrown
- damage to property
- hostage situation
- locking staff in
- threats
- physical violence.

Why violence occurs at work

Violence faced by staff in health and social care arises primarily because the work involves coming into contact with a wide range of people in circumstance which may be difficult. The service users and their relatives may be anxious and worried. Some service users may be predisposed towards violence. Risk of violence is increased in particular circumstances like:

- lone working;

- working after normal working hours;

- working with people who are emotionally or mentally unstable;

- working with people who are under the influence of drinks (alcohol) or drugs;

- working with people under stress;

- working and travelling in the community;

- handling valuables or medication.

Prevention of Violence and aggression at workplace

The following steps help to reduce violence at work;

- Risk assessments of areas and service users to be carried out in accordance with the Health and Safety Policy.

- Organisations to carry out thorough risk assessment of the project or residential care setting.

- Training and information in identified risk areas within the workplace should be provided.

- Individual staff risk assessment for lone workers

- Actions identified by a risk assessment, to be taken as soon as is reasonably possible.

Reporting of violent incidents

- All violent incidents should be reported in accordance with Serious Incident Policy.

- The managers should report immediately if an incident occurs in their specific area.

- You are required to report any incidents of violence, abuse or other incidents that concern you or the service user to the project/residential managers or shift leader.

- All information of reported incidents of violence should be shared as appropriate; especially information on individuals who pose repeated significant risk within the project /residential services should be passed to other organisations in accordance with the confidentiality policy.

Action and advice on dealing with violence and aggression

If as a member of staff you feel you are in danger you should, where possible, leave and summon help immediately.

- You should always make yourself aware of specific precautions to be taken in your workplace, e.g. wearing a personal alarm, keeping the exit route clear and in sight.

- You should never underestimate a threat or be drawn into an argument and never respond in an aggressive manner.

- Up to 90% of communication between individuals is nonverbal, so try to ensure you are not adopting body language that is aggressive, e.g. hands on your hips, or pointing fingers while addressing the service user.

- If you think you have done something to trigger the aggression, consider if you are the best person to deal with the situation or whether someone else could handle the situation more effectively (diffusion model).

- Be aware of the personal space (the length of your outstretched hand in front of yourself defines your personal space); keep your distance. Remember that everyone is different so allow an aggressor room to breathe.

- staff should never put their hands on someone who is angry.

- Remember that many factors, e.g. stresses, frustrations, expectations, levels of learning disabilities, mental health problems can influence how people react to situations; always be aware of as many of these factors as possible.

- Never turn your back on an aggressor, in case of physical attack get away to a place of safety as fast as you can and call for help

- If you witness an aggressive situation think before you get involved. You may be more useful if you call for help.

RECORD KEEPING

What is record keeping?

Record-keeping is the practice of maintaining the records of an organisation from the time they are created up to their eventual disposal and may include evidence of an organisation's activities. For example an organisation providing care services need a high standard of record-keeping to show the delivery of safe and professional care

Daily Records

At the end of each shift you should complete the Daily Log and where relevant, the Medication records and financial transactions with;

- the date, time and signature
- the tasks you performed with and for the service user
- any medication given and any changes in the service user's condition
- information important to colleagues or others involved in the delivery of care
- any accidents and incidents that have happened to the service user or yourself, should be entered in the accident book and Incident report respectively.
- Any financial transactions on behalf of the service user should be recorded. The amount spent and any monies returned with receipts

Record-keeping policy and procedure

The record keeping policy set out the guideline for report writing and daily entries.

- Always:

- o write the date, time, sign each entry;

- o write entries in black ink, which will makes photocopies clearer, if they are required;

- Entries in the daily diaries should be a factual account of each person's day and should include any extraordinary events or incidents that have occurred. They should be written legibly, indelibly, be clear and concise.

- Avoid using 'fuzzy' descriptions. For example, s/he was aggressive/anxious/happy/in a mood. This kind of record entry is open to personal interpretation. Instead try and describe what the person behaved like. For example, s/he paced backwards and forward briskly, vocalising and swearing loudly.

- Records should not include abbreviations and offensive subjective statements.

- If an event (accident/incident) happens that requires an entry in the Accident/Incident book or an 'ABC' chart, write a concise account in the daily entry and then refer the reader to the appropriate book/chart by writing 'see ABC' or 'accident book'. Write in the daily diary as soon as possible after the event; do not leave it until the end of the shift as you may forget the sequence of events.

- If the service user has an appointment with a healthcare professional, state the date, time and who they saw, refer to the GP's records as above. The GP may be asked to fill in their details in the file as well.

- Never deface records or tear pages out.

- Never use Tippex. If you make a mistake, put a single line through the entry, initial it and continue writing.

- Only the name of the service user may be written in full in service user's file. Care worker's initials may be used.

Guidelines to writing daily notes

- Records should be factual, consistent, accurate and in chronological order.

- Records should be written as soon as possible after an event has occurred using reflective practice, providing current information on the care/condition of the service user.

- Records should provide clear evidence of the care planned, the decisions made, the care given and the information shared.

- Records should be written in such a manner that any alterations or additions are dated, timed using the 24-hour clock and signed with the author's name printed alongside when making the first entry and include the author's position.

- Records should not include abbreviations, jargon, meaningless phrases, irrelevant speculation and offensive subjective statements.

- Records should be readable on any photocopies.

- Records should be clearly written and legible.

All records should be written objectively stating what you have actually done. Never assume or write what you think about the service user. These records are legal documents that could be used in a court of law. You should complete them accurately, concisely and legibly with a black ball pen.

Why organisations keep daily records?

It is important to keep daily record in a service because;

- Complete service based records provide current, valid and appropriate information for evidence based practice

- It promotes continuity of care and ensures consistency in support;

- It demonstrates high standards of care and evidence of care being given, the intervention by professional practitioners and service users' responses;

- It enhances communication and sharing of information between care workers and other professionals;

- Daily records help to protect service users and care workers, by keeping accurate records of the action taken and the care given;

- It allows deterioration/progress in service users' condition to be detected at an early stage;

- It provides the chronology of events and the reasons for any decisions made e.g. why 'PRN' medication was prescribed

- It enables all members of the multidisciplinary team to care for the service user regardless of what stages they have reached in the care process;

- Good records can be used in a court of law;

- For monitoring and review purposes to ensure compliance with standards, legislation and good practice guidance.

Accident/Incident Report

If during the course of your work an accident occurs to you or the service user or other household members during a visit, complete the Accident Book or in case of an incident complete an Incident Report and submit to your manager or supervisor. Ensure that you verbally report an accident immediately to your manager in advance of your written report.

Storage and transportation of records

- Records should not be stored in an area that other service users, members of the public or unauthorised members of staff can gain access to them.

- Where records are stored in areas that do not have 24-hour staff presence, then they should be stored in an area that can be securely locked when the premises are unstaffed.

- If records need to be transported from one organisation to another, it is the responsibility of the staff processing the request to ensure that at no point could the records be accessed by unauthorised individuals.

- It is staff responsibility to ensure that any records are stored safely and securely whilst in transit.

Summary

Remember… to avoid complications in the review process keep your records thorough and updated. *If it's not recorded, it did not happen!*